Reverse

Diabetes

The Ultimate Beginner's Diet Guide To Reversing Diabetes - A Guide to Finally Cure, Lower & Control Your Blood Sugar

By *Louise Jiannes*

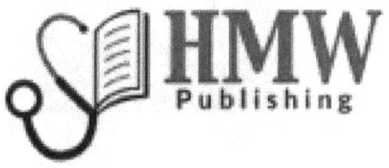

For more great books visit:

HMWPublishing.com

Get another book for Free

I want to thank you for purchasing this book and offer you another book (just as long and valuable as this book), "Health & Fitness Mistakes You Don't Know You're Making", completely free.

Visit the link below to signup and receive it:

www.hmwpublishing.com/gift

In this book, I will break down the most common health & fitness mistakes, you are probably committing right now, and I will reveal how you can easily get in the best shape of your life!

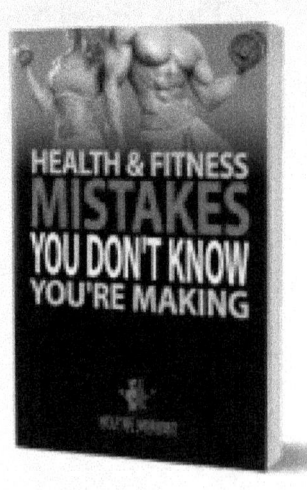

In addition to this valuable gift, you will also have an opportunity to get our new books for free, enter giveaways, and receive other valuable emails from me. Again, visit the link to sign up:

www.hmwpublishing.com/gift

Table of Contents

Introduction 2

Chapter 1 – Why Diabetics Struggle with Weight Loss 5

    Bad diet 5
    Antioxidants 6
    Insulin 9
    Belly Fat 10
    Fatty liver 13
    Parasites 14
    How to beat these powerful mechanisms? 16
    Glucose management 18
    Fasting 20
    Physical activities 21

Chapter 2 – The Diabetic Weight Loss Challenge: Where to Start? 25

    Why do you gain weight? 26
    Different points of view 27

Chapter 3 – How to Avoid Insulin Resistance and Manage Diabetes Naturally 30

    Symptoms and Conditions of Insulin Resistance 31
    Causes of Diabetes and Insulin Resistance 32
    Diet and nutrition for Type II diabetes/Insulin Resistance 33
    Supplemental nutrients for insulin resistance 34
    Supplemental botanicals 35
    Lifestyle protocol 36

Exercise protocol 37

Chapter 4 – Insulin Resistance Diet Guideline 39

Type II Diabetes Definition and Facts 39

What is Type II Diabetes? 41

What Types of Foods are Recommended for a Type II Diabetes? 42

What Types of Carbohydrates are Recommended? 44

Starchy vegetables and grains 45

Non-starchy vegetables 47

What Types of Fat are Recommended? 49

What Types of Protein are Recommended? 50

What Types of Meal Plans or Diet are Recommended for People with Type II Diabetes? 51

Vegetarian or Vegan Diets 52

American Diabetes Association (ADA) Diabetes Diet 53

Paleo Diet 54

Mediterranean Diet 55

5 Diabetes Superfoods to Eat 56

Foods to be Avoided in Type II Diabetes Meal Plan 59

Alcohol and Type II Diabetes 61

Healthier Choices When Eating Out 62

Complications of Type II Diabetes 63

Conclusion 64

INTRODUCTION

I want to thank you and congratulate you for downloading the *"Reverse Diabetes"* book. Diabetes is among the most common ailments in the modern times. People across the globe suffer from this disease and so they undergo treatment. As a matter of fact, it has become a lifestyle disease, and most of the time, it is hereditary or chronic disease. Because of this, this disease has become unavoidable each single day, and it goes beyond control. Those who suffer from diabetes either lose weight excessively, become overweight. In connection with this, people suffering from overweight issues most commonly have to go on diet in order to retain a healthy status and control the disease.

Losing weight and dieting is among the primary key to have good health. Having the right diet means developing a better health. To be able to lose weight and retain a balanced physique, patients must undertake particular important steps. Included in these things are proper diet, physical exercises, and an overall balanced lifestyle. When you have a relatively lower weight, you will be healthier and will have a better heart too. Thus, being in the right weight is very essential for a diabetic person. First of all, mental preparation is very important when choosing the right diet and building commitment into better health.

It is important to have an understanding about diabetes, the importance of losing weight, and how to do so. All answers can be found in this book. Thanks again for purchasing this book, I hope you enjoy it!

Also, before you get started, I recommend you **joining our email newsletter** to receive updates on any upcoming new book releases or promotions. You can sign-up for free, and as a bonus, you will receive a free gift. Our "*Health & Fitness Mistakes You Don't Know You're Making*" book! This book has been written to demystify, expose the top do's and don'ts and to finally equip you with the information you need to get in the best shape of your life. Due to the overwhelming amount of mis-information and lies told by magazines and self-proclaimed "gurus", it's becoming harder and harder to get reliable information to get in shape. As opposed to having to go through dozens of biased, unreliable and untrustworthy sources to get your health & fitness information. Everything you need to help you has been broken down in this book for you to easily follow and to immediately get results to achieve your desired fitness goals in the shortest amount of time.

Once again, to join our free email newsletter and to receive a free copy of this valuable book, please visit the link and signup now: www.hmwpublishing.com/gift

Chapter 1 – Why Diabetics Struggle with Weight Loss

Among the most perplexing problems faced by people with diabetes is losing weight. Some doctors insist that it is just a simple way of consuming less sugar and fewer calories than burning them. However, most diabetic patients are asking that there is more to it, for the reason that when they do the same thing and eat the same food like that of the non-diabetic people, they do not get results, whereas their friends who do not have diabetes have been dropping pound after pound. It does not work to go on fad diets and taking diet products, and even exercise does not show results. The struggling diabetic people are right – there is more to it than just cutting calories.

Bad diet

The cause of diabetes is when you eat unhealthy food, and the key to regaining control is through proper nutrition. However, it is the lousy diet that placed many conditions in place that should be understood to be able to win the weight loss war. Several interrelated events bring a significant contribution to making weight loss for diabetes hard. Firstly, it is essential to see where the problem is originated. You can then investigate when and how the information may lead to reversing the problem.

Containing sweets, fats, prepared foods, dairy products, and foods with high glycemic index – years of bad diet can cause inflammation. A detailed and complete explanation of how inflammation causes diabetes can be found in this chapter. Some of the reasons for diabetes are due to space limitations and gross over-simplification. Pro-inflammatory substances or pro-oxidants are used commonly by the body to combat infection and disease through our immune system. They have many significant roles to play in the body, including breathing and digestion.

Antioxidants

Most commonly, antioxidants are used by our body for

controlling these processes. Nonetheless, years of bad diet can cause the immune system to lose the capability to shut down, which has low antioxidants characteristically. The immune system will then start attacking the healthy cells that produce severe damage. In the Type II diabetes, the insulin-producing cells or beta cells, are destroyed. Here, many cells are damaged, as it sets up a condition called insulin resistance, which occurs when the cells of the body are not able to communicate appropriately when using insulin for burning and up-taking glucose.

When your body digests food, more specifically carbohydrates, it will be converted to glucose, which is distributed all over the body in the liver's bloodstream. The liver is commonly the one controlling fat levels. When there are very high levels of sugar in the blood, due to the diet, the liver then will not be able to process it all. It will then start filling the cells with sacs of converted glucose for storage called triglycerides, placing the excess in the belly fat.

The vital organs, brain, and muscle tissue are relying on glucose, which is providing energy to function. Because these organs are using glucose, the liver will be placing more in the bloodstream to replace it. In a perfect world, the tissues and organs use it in an efficient way, and in proportion to the amount that foods produced. Insulin resistance decreases the amount of glucose that is stored and absorbed by the muscle tissue and organs. In addition to that, the fact that most people with diabetes lead a sedentary lifestyle, which means that they are getting minimal amounts of exercise and it results in having less glucose to burn.

When type II diabetes impairs the body, the cells are not using as much glucose. The body will sense that the glucose levels build up in the bloodstream, so it is instructing the pancreas for more insulin to be released. Now, the body has high levels of glucose and high levels of insulin in the bloodstream. Insulin is a hormone that has many functions to perform, in addition to allowing the cells to absorb glucose. It also tries to eliminate the excess glucose from your bloodstream vigorously, and so it places it in storage as fat. As soon as it is in the storage, the insulin will be blocking the process to break this fat down to remove it from storage.

Insulin

The presence of high insulin levels in the blood will cause unnecessary retention of water in the body – one factor to gain weight. This is the central aspect of beating diabetic obesity, and with this, insulin regulation is of great importance. Furthermore, insulin acts on the brain, promoting the cravings that lead to eating more and on the liver manufacturing more fats. The liver functions to remove insulin from the bloodstream. Nonetheless, insulin is the cause of fats to be deposited in the liver, preventing the liver to remove insulin from the blood. Those who have belly fats are storing too much fat in their livers, which is known as fatty liver disease, preventing the liver from eliminating insulin. Thus, the levels of insulin will continue to rise higher and higher, which may bring a significant contribution to more abdominal obesity and heart attacks.

Additionally, the fat in abdominal area functions differently as compared to that of the fat in other parts of the body like hips. The flow of blood from belly fats goes directly to the liver. The flow of blood from different fatty areas like hips will go through general circulation of the body. Belly fat has efficient supply of blood and has more receptors for a stress hormone, called cortisol. The levels of cortisol vary from the day, but it is going to rise and remain high if your body is under stress. High levels of cortisol and stress promote fat deposits in the belly area because there are more cortisol receptors there.

High levels of cortisol chronically kill brain neurons, and interfere with the neurotransmitters like serotonin and dopamine. These are neurotransmitters in a good mood, which lead to feeling more stressed and depressed. Depression is ubiquitous in people with diabetes, and this will add to the problem because depression is causing a stress kind of reaction in the body. In other words, depression will promote belly fat development.

Belly Fat

Belly fat is a characteristic of diabetes, meaning, people with diabetes will be prone having belly fat. Central obesity, or belly fat, is significantly associated with higher rates of cardiovascular disease, and many kinds of cancer too. Heredity has a role to play in your overall body types, such as a pear-shaped body or an apple-typed body. There is about 25 to 55% of the tendency of developing the most dangerous diseases that are associated with abdominal fat. The remaining is lifestyle. Belly fats do several things as it builds up. It, first of all, stops hormone leptin production, which would curb appetite. Another thing about this is that it causes increase in insulin resistance, which will lead to apparent consequences. The cells are using less glucose, and so the body would produce more insulin, and then, the fat will go into storage.

Fat storage is the way of the body to follow ancient mechanisms, which are designed to protect your body in lean times. The body learns to take advantage of the excellent opportunities in order to prepare for the bad times. The body will then convert the glucose to triglycerides and glycogen, which are useful methods to store energy. When the liver cells are filled with triglyceride fat sacs, the function of the liver is going to be impaired. It will not be able to process fats efficiently. It will run out of room for storing more fat quickly, and when the organs and tissues of the body do not use as much, the liver will just put all these in storage as belly fat.

The number of fat cells that we have will be identified at birth. The numbers will stay constant unless the fat cells become full, and when it does, the cells are going to divide in making new fat cells. The new cells will then remain all over the balance of the person's life. On the other hand, when you undergo a successful diet, you are reducing the size of fat cells in your body. These fat cells are fed by our blood vessels in belly area. Every fat cell is in contact with a minimum of one capillary. The supply of blood is providing support for your metabolism. The flow of blood varies upon body weight, as well as your overall nutritional condition. The blood vessels are going to increase when it demands highly for glucose or during fasting, resulting in rising blood pressure. The heart has to directly work much harder in order to supply the additional vessels.

Fatty liver

A liver with many cells that is full of triglyceride sacs is called a fatty liver or non-alcoholic fatty liver disease (NAFLD). Any individual with diabetes who has an excellent amount of belly fat is more likely to have a fatty liver, which develops early in progress due to high levels of triglycerides in your bloodstream. The second stage of your fatty liver is called the non-alcoholic steatohepatitis (NASH). This means that it is not caused by consuming alcohol, but similar. It poses the same damage as that of the hepatitis disease. Cell oxidation starts occurring as caused by cell damage. Furthermore, the 3rd stage of fatty liver is cirrhosis, and it is a severe and dangerous condition.

Fatty liver in stage I is not particularly dangerous, and it can be cured with proper treatment. Doctors will be conducting a biopsy to identify how much fat is there and if there is any scarring present too. A biopsy is seldom undertaken because the medical industry is not able to agree on how it must be interpreted. The signs and symptoms of NAFLD are non-existent, non-descript, and it mimics the symptoms of other diseases. Specific blood tests can display the presence of particular liver enzymes that are usual in hepatitis, which are signifying the signs and presence of the NASH. The fatty liver is a severe complication in the process of losing weight.

Parasites

These parasites stall weight loss efforts implicitly, and these are common in people with diabetes as compared to those who do not have, because they are in a weakened condition. Unfortunately, western medical doctors do not have enough training in noticing the presence of parasites. There are only a few people, who are trained in testing for these conditions. Among the most common tests have a meager rate of accuracy. Drugs that treat parasites are rarely used for the reason that they have a small range of effectiveness. More than a hundred of common species are found in humans, with treatments being particular to specie. Parasites can escape diagnosis in as many as 70 chronic diseases, and now, they are believed to be instrumental in the development process of many chronic illnesses.

When there are parasites present, the patients will not succeed in weight loss process. Counting or eliminating carbohydrates, reducing portion sizes, or doing vigorous exercise is not going to produce results. Parasites will inflame the lining of digestive tract, and thus, slow the absorption of nutrient. Eventually, they spread to all parts of the body including your vital organs, and hence, disrupting the regulation of blood sugar, hormonal balance, and altering the metabolism. The parasites eat nutrients you ingest, or they may eat the host, leaving it with empty calories. This triggers overconsumption of foods and cravings, and then, they would take over control in your body.

Moreover, parasites release toxins that are overloading the liver and kidneys. Your weakened condition will lead to further reductions in the metabolism, hindering the maintenance of your beneficial flora in the intestinal tract. Because of this, there can be overproduction of yeasts. Overdeveloping yeasts will result in developing gas, allergies, and bloating. Their acids can damage the organs and break down the muscle tissue, and may also cause the sluggish central nervous system. The body reacts to increased levels of acid by producing fat cells in order to store the acid, and thereby, it removes it from your system. Fat cells can be produced when you have lower metabolism.

How to beat these powerful mechanisms?

The great news here is that these days, the reasons why it is hard to lose weight is more apparent. So, how will you be able to beat these powerful mechanisms? Begin by eliminating the parasites. Assume that they are present because there is a significant possibility that they are present. It is important to modify your diet to eat only low glycemic index foods. Stop yourself from eating foods that are high in oxidants, more mainly processed foods. These processed foods include any meals in a can or box with ingredients that you cannot pronounce, or unknown to you as to why that particular ingredient is there.

Then, assume that you have a fatty liver, because you may

have to some extent. It will be a hard part. The most success comes from merging several methods. Exercise and fasting are effective in breaking the cycles and burning liver fat. However, it needs to be done in the right manner. If kidney or liver damage is present, consult your doctor. One alternative to fasting is, to begin with very light and low glycemic index meals every day, rather than having 3 large meals daily. This will decrease the glucose spikes that exacerbate the process.

It is of great importance that you change your diet. Processed foods are considered poison to people with diabetes, and it can't be pointed out enough. The processed flour is terrible for those who have diabetes. Also, sodas have high phosphoric acid and oxidants. You can drink tea as alternative. You should even stop drinking coffee. Do not cook foods at high temperature, or do not microwave your foods. It also means that broiling and grilling are out. Take quality multivitamins every day.

Glucose management

Managing your glucose can be improved if your levels of sodium are maintained and if the levels of fiber are kept high. Sodium can slow the insulin response, and this means that higher levels of sodium can be an advantage for those with hypoglycemia. High levels of sodium will prevent a fast fall and rise in your insulin levels, and thus, decreasing the blood sugar that is usually experienced with hypoglycemia. Together with vitamin C, sodium and biotin are among essential factors to reduce level of erratic glucose, even between meals.

Aside from that, chromium, manganese, and niacinamide/niacin help in controlling glucose response and the liver's storage of glycogen. Vitamin C, vitamin B6, and potassium are all helpful in stabilizing or interfering with glucose management, depending on whether you are prone to hyperglycemia or hypoglycemia. The lower amount of glucose is recommended for those who are likely to hypoglycemia, and higher amount of glucose is recommended for people who are prone to hyperglycemia.

Alternately, high amount of potassium helps in reducing chromium and manganese. Also, high amount of vitamin C is lowering manganese and stimulating insulin. Vitamin B6 then helps in stimulating potassium and magnesium, but it reduces the manganese. It may be complicated, so it is important to keep in mind that too much sodium in your diet will never be a good thing.

Stop eating honey, candies, all kinds of sodas, cereals, cakes and bakery foods, sugar, syrups, sucrose, dextrose, donuts, fruit juices, fructose, maltose, overripe fruits, or any substances that end in "use." Stop intake of all artificial sweeteners, except the Stevia. Most bakery foods contain synthetic additives, together with the processed flour, both of which have high oxidative. Another important thing is taking exercises in order to maximize the glucose being burnt in tissues. You can do power walking for around 45 minutes every day, resulting in 300 calories burn-up daily. Doing other muscle exercises is a great help. You should alternate the exercise program and fasting with non-fast exercise programs with a span of 3 to 5 days every program.

Fasting

Depending on your health conditions, try to select between a glass of juice or a glass of water to start the fast. You will notice that the water fasting feel like it is working more. Primarily, due to the lower calories/energy, it contains. It is recommended not to lose weight too fast because it may damage your liver. Most people would lose around three to five pounds after their first few days of losing weight, and additional three to five pounds on the next day. This is going to level off at one pound every day after dropping several pounds initially. It is required not to lose weight during the non-fasting phase. Then, repeat the cycle.

On the next chapters of this book, we will discuss several programs for losing weight to reverse diabetes. The most aggressive of the weight loss programs for reversing diabetes is a 30-day fasting, which is going to detox the whole body too completely. It is known well for releasing toxins that are present since birth. Fasting is safe and effective. When you exercise a muscle, it will not remove the fat over specific exercised muscles. The only way for you to decrease a belly fat is by losing weight overall, and any kinds of exercise will be a great help in accomplishing that. The quickest way of burning belly fat is through a combination of aerobic exercise, weight training, and a modified diet. Keep in your mind that increased muscle mass through working out which will help in improving your body weight because of fat loss.

Physical activities

It is beneficial for people with diabetes are doing physical activities. This will also lower your blood glucose levels. However, it can make the levels go too low, which causes hypoglycemia for around 24 hours afterward. For diabetic people who take insulin or those who seek oral medications that increase the production of insulin, fasting through a snack may be necessary if the level of glucose goes below 100 mg/dL. It can be helpful for avoiding hypoglycemia to adjust the doses of your medication before doing any physical activity. For other diabetic people, you may need to consult your doctor while you are on the progressive programs.

A snack can avert hypoglycemia, given that it's a portion of food with lowered glycemic index. There may be necessary extra checks in blood glucose, more particularly 2 hours after a strenuous exercise. Have an increased emphasis to maintain the blood sugar levels. Hold them closer to normal. In the insulin resistance, it will decrease the amount of extra insulin in your bloodstream. If you are insulin dependent, if you are someone with Type I diabetes, you should avoid taking more insulin as compared to what is necessary for maintaining control. Many people who have diabetes assume that having more insulin as compared to what you need is not necessarily a bad thing.

It is a critical phase requiring lots of focus and testing. The combination of having lower insulin, vigorous exercise, lower levels of glucose enable the body to start burning the liver fat quickly. There are about 12 to 16 hours necessary in order to draw fat from your liver, and but with exercise, you can increase your metabolism. On the other hand, understanding the metabolism is a great help, because the rate of your metabolism will change the process. Doing exercises can reduce the levels of stress. If high stress is a problem, try doing activities that reduce stress, such as meditation and deep breathing. Do not forget to take antioxidant supplements during the fasting process.

Omega-3 fats can help in reducing the output of epinephrine, another stress hormone. Consider around 40000IU of fish oil 2x a day, but do not overdose on fish oil because your body will be producing significant amounts of free radicals, which will also require vast amounts of antioxidants in order to be controlled. Make sure you will consume 100% of daily requirements of minerals and vitamins. It is highly recommended to modify your diet and learn what you should and should not eat. Also, take a right quality multivitamin each day. Control your glucose levels and manager the levels of sodium. On the other hand, it is also important to manage your insulin levels, handle stress, exercise every day vigorously, consider several fasting techniques, and eliminate the possibility of parasite infestation. Learn about foods and diabetes as much as possible, and learn how to maintain and cleanse all the vital organs.

It may appear to be lots of hard work. Well, it indeed is, but it is usually for people with diabetes, who did not experience any success when dieting. The key to reversing diabetes is total control and improved health through weight loss. The next chapter discusses where to start on your diabetic weight loss challenge.

Chapter 2 – The Diabetic Weight Loss Challenge: Where to Start?

People with diabetes are highly advised to lose weight. However, for most, it is easily said than done. Diabetic people are encouraged to eat the right food, with several foods to be avoided, including foods with high sodium content and high saturated fats. It is hard to change the old habits, but it is also important to exercise more and eat less. This is something that we know but we do not do.

Unless the person with diabetes is provided with a more detailed meal planning guide, it is left for him/her to work out on their approach and different ways to attain a weight loss goal, finding exactly they need to eat and how much to eat. Losing weight for a diabetic person can be a complicated process, especially for identifying a target weight and the appropriate foods, so if possible, the person with diabetes should request for advice and a tailored diet plan.

Why do you gain weight?

The reason why you are gaining weight is that more food is consumed as compared to what you needed in order to stay alive. Your body will convert any excess food and store it in the form of fat. As seen in calories, some foods are more abundant as compared to others weight for weight. Fats provide more calories per gram as compared to those with non-fats. Your body needs fat, just as it needs carbohydrates and protein, but it is important to eat less fatty foods.

There are ratios of proteins, fats, and carbohydrates established by nutritionists that are considered appropriate in order to maintain good health for the general population. Carbohydrates are supplying most of the necessary glucose by our body cells for energy. Even though when there are no carbohydrates, the body will be using protein to make the required glucose. The glucose is the problem that diabetic people face because their body can't control the glucose content as that of the people without diabetes.

In the case for people with diabetes, too much glucose is not going to your body cells that require it, but it remains in the bloodstream for a long time, which it poses harm and damage. Carbohydrates have many categories, as classified by the content's complexity to their sugar-containing molecules, wherein there are lots of many. In line with this, the more complicated they are, the longer it will take for the digestive system of the body's chemical actions to break them down into glucose.

Furthermore, the longer time there is to do this will diminish the peak of increased load of glucose in the bloodstream, which may occur after you eat. To people with diabetes, this condition of elevated blood glucose lasts longer as compared to what it does for those who do not have diabetes – it is a problem. Carbohydrates are providing the required glucose, which is the cause of diabetes. This is what diabetes is all about. High blood sugar for a too long time will result in lots of other health problems.

Different points of view

There are 2 conflicting schools of thought about the ratio and amount of carbohydrates, as compared to other essential nutrients, which must be consumed by those with diabetic. Here, the approach to reversing diabetes followed by successful and well-known medical practitioners is by keeping the ratio of carbohydrates, the primary source of glucose, and the low end of scale as compared to the fat and protein content. With this, it is recommended to leverage the effectiveness of low carb diet, supported by particular vitamins and dietary supplements, and exercising.

To help determine complex carbs, you can check in the glycemic index – providing a numerical rating of foods that contain carbohydrates. Lower carb diets help people with diabetes to control their high glucose problems. However, in their view, though it produces the correct results, it is hard to follow for any length of time. Maybe you would decide on that, but the National Diabetic Associations have made a little effort in making awareness to people with diabetes about what the lower carb diets would be able to accomplish.

Comprehensively outstanding meal planning for people with diabetes is available for both high carb and low carb advocates. Weight loss and diabetic weight loss program is a dangerous process and that you should discuss it with a doctor. This is the responsibility and right of the diabetic patient to decide on which route they should follow. However, it is wise if you would confide in, discussing the merits of their choices with their doctor. Much management and control of the diabetic condition are left to the patient, and there are required monitoring levels of glucose in the blood each day. There are also times when the control is reduced many times a day.

The next chapter will help you understand how you can avoid insulin resistance and manage your diabetes naturally.

Chapter 3 – How to Avoid Insulin Resistance and Manage Diabetes Naturally

Insulin resistance is when the cell, more specifically the muscle, liver, and fat cells, is not being responsive on your insulin receptor site. With this, your body will continue to add more and more insulin for storing fat. Through time, the pancreas will be giving up, and this results in insulin resistance or Type II diabetes. In this diabetes level, your body does not make enough insulin or the cells will be resistant to insulin, which causes too much sugar to stay in your blood.

A fasting level of your blood glucose, higher than 100 to 125 mg/dL, it will not be an indication of diabetes. However, it may become a determinant of insulin resistance, which is beyond the reasonable levels. The maximum range of serum glucose is between 80 and 95. Fasting serum insulin levels need to be below 10. One of the most potent anti-aging and diabetes-reversing strategies for a healthy new you, is to control your insulin levels utilizing diet plan, together with exercise, several lifestyle modifications, proper nutrition, and supplements. This is a must for your longevity, fat loss, vitality, and overall health.

Symptoms and Conditions of Insulin Resistance

- Hypertension

- Inability to focus and brain fogginess

- Low HDL levels

- Elevated triglycerides

- Type II diabetes

- Excess fat around your scapula area or midsection

- Intestinal bloating

- Fatigue and sleepiness

When your glucose builds up in your blood rather than going into the cells, it can cause problems, including

- Obesity

- Higher risk of Alzheimer's disease

- Through time, high levels of blood glucose can damage your kidneys, heart, eyes, or nerves

Causes of Diabetes and Insulin Resistance

- Lack of quality sleep

- Drinking fruit juices and soft drinks

- Sedentary lifestyle

- Altered hormonal levels and stress

- Skipping meals, calorie restriction, crap diet of microwaved, boxed, or canned foods, diet pills, and fast foods.

- Decreased lipolytic enzymes and increased lipogenic enzymes

Diet and nutrition for Type II diabetes/ Insulin Resistance

- Small mini meals 5 to 7 times per day. Include protein and smart fats in every meal

- Get rid of all canned, boxed, and microwavable foods

- Enabled fruits in moderation, including berries, limes, tomatoes, grapefruit, avocados, and lemons

- Increase protein and cutting carbs. Eat a diet of non-starchy vegetables, organic proteins, and fats

- Get rid of all grains, fast-acting sugars, refined carbs, and dairy products. Avoid soft drinks, starchy vegetables, juices, and high glycemic fruits. Also avoid hydrogenated fats like caffeine, alcohol, and tobacco

- Sweeten foods with stevia instead of sugar. Stevia does not increase blood sugar

- Avoid Nutra Sweet and Aspartame products, agave syrup, and HFCS, because they can trigger obesity and diabetes

- Lime and lemon juice can decrease the insulin index of meals because of the flavonoids

Supplemental nutrients for insulin resistance

- Fiber

- Resveratrol

- R-alpha lipoic acid

- Potassium, zinc, and magnesium deficiencies result to insulin resistance

- GlucoBalance

- Vitamin D

- 7-keto DHEA

- Bio-glycozyme forte

- Improve insulin sensitivity with glutathione, CoQ, L-Arginine, Taurine, and L-Carnitine

- Silymarin

- ADHS

- Chromium

- Omega-3 fish oil with 400 IU

Supplemental botanicals

- Tea like Pau d' Arco, Fenugreek, green tea, Burdock, and Astragalus

- Banaba tree extract

- Gymnema Sylvestre

- Bitter gourd

- Grape seed extract

- Cinnamon

Lifestyle protocol

- Get fasting insulin levels and serum glucose

- Rule out the heavy metal burdens, pesticides, and other inoculations and xenobiotics

- Make sure you have a healthy gut flora. Consider a Comprehensive Digestive Stool Analysis (CDSA)

- Take care of your eyes. This is because diabetes is a primary cause of being blind. This can result to retinopathy and other eye problems like cataracts

- It is essential to monitor your blood glucose levels at least twice per day and before you eat meals. If you are doing exercise, you should test your level of glucose more frequently

- Rule out your food allergies with decreased or increased blood sugar

- Go to bed at 10 PM and get up no earlier than 6 AM. This is because lack of sleep disturbs glucose metabolism, blood pressure, memory, lipid profile, immune system, and androgen production.

Exercise protocol

- You should never underestimate the power of being active, from a short 5-minute walk to 45-minute training sessions for strength, this all counts down to eliminating and reducing pre-diabetes syndrome or insulin resistance.

- Compared to aerobic steady state exercises, strength training is much superior in preventing obesity as well as in improving the insulin resistance. The constant aerobic state exercises the cortisol levels which the insulin levels.

- Start some exercise routine. A simple walking is excellent for diabetes. An everyday 3mph brisk walking can decrease the risk of diabetes by 50%.

Chapter 4 – Insulin Resistance Diet Guideline

Type II diabetes or Insulin resistance is a condition where your cells are not able to use glucose or blood sugar for energy in an efficient way. This happens when the cells are not any more sensitive to the insulin and with this, your blood sugar will get too high gradually.

Type II Diabetes Definition and Facts

Type II diabetes has problems with getting enough glucose into the cells. When the sugar is not able to get where it is supposed to be, it will result to having increased blood sugar levels in your bloodstream, which may lead to complications like nerve, cardiovascular disease, kidney, and eye damage. Foods to eat the right diet for a person with type II diabetes include complex carbs like whole wheat, fruits, beans, brown rice, oatmeal, lentils, vegetables, quinoa, and beans. Foods that must be avoided in type II diabetes include simple carbs that are processed, like pasta, cookies, flour, white bread, sugar IQ, and pastries. Foods that have low glycemic index will cause a modest rise in your blood sugar and so this is better option for diabetic people. Good glycemic control can be helpful in preventing long-term complications of insulin resistance.

Fats IQ does not have much direct effect on your blood sugar but it can be of great use for you in slowing carbs absorption. Protein is providing steady energy with small impact on the blood sugar. It keeps the blood sugar stable and it is helpful to your sugar cravings and feeling full after eating. Foods packed with protein to east include legumes, dairy, lean meats, beans, peas, poultry, seafood, eggs, and tofu. Added in the five diabetes superfoods IQ are white balsamic vinegar, lentils, wild salmon, chia seeds, and cinnamon. Furthermore, healthy diabetes IQ meal plans include limited red meat and processed sugars, and lots of vegetables. Diet recommendations for those with type II diabetes IQ include a vegan or vegetarian diet, which emphasizes doing exercise, Mediterranean diet, and the Paleo diet.

Guidelines on what diabetic people should eat include eating low glycemic index carbs, more particularly from vegetables, consuming proteins and fats from plant sources. Foods that you should not eat if you have insulin resistance include processed carbs, high-fat dairy products, artificial sweeteners, high-fat animal products, sodas, high fructose corn syrup, trans fats, refined sugars, and any highly processed foods.

What is Type II Diabetes?

Type II diabetes or insulin resistance occurs through time, involving problems about getting enough sugar or glucose into your body cells. The cells are using sugar for energy or fuel. Glucose or sugar has been the ideal fuel for brain cells and muscle cells, but it requires insulin in order to transport it into cells and be useful. When the levels of insulin are low, with the sugar not being able to get into the cells where it is supposed to be, it leads to increased blood sugar levels.

As time passes by, the cells will start developing resistance to insulin, which will then require your pancreas to make more and more insulin to move the sugar into the cells, but more sugar is still left in your blood. Eventually, the pancreas wears out and may not anymore be able to secrete enough insulin for moving the sugar to the cells for energy.

What Types of Foods are Recommended for a Type II Diabetes?

Diabetic people should follow the dietary guidelines. Eating the recommended amount of foods from the 5 food groups will provide you with the necessary nutrients in order to be healthy and prevent chronic diseases like heart disease and obesity.

A diabetic meal plan may follow several different patterns and have a variable ratio of proteins, carbs, and fats. The consumed carbohydrates should be low glycemic index and should mainly come from vegetables. The absorbed proteins and fat should primarily come from plant sources.

To help you in managing your diabetes, it is recommended to eat regular meals and spread them evenly across the day. Eat a diet that is lower in fat, specifically saturated fat. If you are taking diabetes tablets or insulin, you may need to have it between-meal snacks.

It is important to know that everyone's needs are not the same. All people who have diabetes need to see an accredited dietician in conjunction with their diabetes team for individualized advice.

What Types of Carbohydrates are Recommended?

Carbohydrates are the primary food that raises blood sugar. Glycemic load and glycemic index are the scientific names used for measuring the impact of carbohydrates on the blood sugar. Foods that have low glycemic index are modestly raising blood sugar and thereby, they are better options for diabetic people. The primary factors that identify the glycemic load of a meal or specific food are the amount of protein, fiber, and fats that it contains.

The difference between glycemic load and glycemic index is that the glycemic index is a standardized measurement while the glycemic load accounts for a real-life size. Like for instance, the glycemic index of one bowl of peas is 68, but the glycemic load is only 16. The lower glycemic level, the better. If you preferred to the glycemic index, you would think that peas have been built like a bad option, but the truth is that you would not be eating a hundred grams of peas. With a regular portion size, the peas would have a healthy glycemic load, and it can be an excellent source of protein.

Carbs can be classified as either simple sugars or complex carbs. The complex carbohydrates or low glycemic load foods are in their entire food form and this includes additional nutrients like vitamins, fiber, and smaller amounts of fats and proteins. These extra nutrients will slow down glucose absorption, keeping the blood sugar levels more stable. Some of the low glycemic index or complex carbs foods to include in your Type II diabetes diet plan are whole wheat, fruits, lentils, brown rice, vegetables, quinoa, beans, and steel-cut oatmeal.

Starchy vegetables and grains

Whole grains like quinoa, oatmeal, and brown rice are excellent sources of nutrients and fiber, and they have a low glycemic index, which makes them suitable choices for food. The labels of processed foods make it confusing to understand the whole grains. For instance, the whole wheat bread is made in various ways and there are some that do not have that much difference from white bread in its glycemic index. The same holds true for the whole grain pasta. Whole grains have less impact on the blood sugar since there is lower glycemic load. Select whole grains that are still in their grain forms, such as quinoa and brown rice, or you may look at the fiber content on the nutritional label of the particular food. A good whole grain bread has 3+ g. of fiber in every slice.

Starchy vegetables are excellent sources of nutrients such as vitamin C, and they are high in carbs as compared to green leafy vegetables; however, they are lower in carbs as compared to refined grains. Diabetic people can eat them in moderation. Some of the starchy vegetables are corn, potatoes, squash, and other root vegetables. These foods are best eaten in smaller portions, like one cup, as part of your diabetic meal plant for plant-based fat and protein.

Non-starchy vegetables

Diabetic people can eat non-starchy vegetables in abundance, like the green vegetables, because they have limited impact on your blood sugar, and they have lots of health benefits. Most people can eat more vegetable. We all need as little as 5 servings every day. One great option is fresh vegetables, and they are most commonly the tastiest option. Frozen vegetables have just as many nutrients and vitamins IQ, as they usually are frozen within hours of harvesting.

To ensure that there are no addition

sweeteners or fats in sauces, check the label on the frozen vegetables. If you are a fan of vegetables on their own, you may try to prepare them with some dried or fresh herbs, vinaigrette dressing, or olive oil. One good way of getting all your nutrients is by consuming a rainbow of colors with your vegetables.

The high glycemic load or simple carbs foods, or foods that are not part of the diet plan for type II diabetes are processed foods. These foods do not contain other nutrients that can help in slowing down sugar absorption and hence, they are raising blood sugar quickly. Lots of simple carbs foods are known as the white foods. Some of the simple carb foods that should be avoided in the insulin resistance diet plan are white potatoes, cookies, white bread, white pasta, pineapples, watermelon, pastries, sugar, sweets, flour, soft drinks, and breakfast cereals.

What Types of Fat are Recommended?

Fats have small direct effect on the blood sugar. However, as part of a meal, they have a great use in slowing down carbohydrates absorption. Also, fats have effects on health that are unrelated to glucose. Plant-based fats like nuts, avocado, olive oil, and seeds are associated with lower cardiovascular disease risk. Animal meat fats are increasing the risk of cardiovascular disease. Nevertheless, dairy and the particularly fermented dairy products like yogurt are decreasing the disease risk. Also, fat contributes to feelings of satiety and they have a role to play in managing carbohydrate cravings and overeating. A part of healthy fats, such as avocado on the whole grain toast, is more robust and more satisfying as compared to jam on white toast.

What Types of Protein are Recommended?

There is a slow, steady energy provided by protein, which has small effect on your blood sugar. Protein, particularly the plant-based protein, needs always to be a part of your meal plan or snack. This nutrient will not only keep your blood sugar stable, but it is also helpful in your sugar cravings and feeling full after eating satiety. Furthermore, protein may come from either plant or animal sources, but animal sources are also familiar sources of unhealthy saturated fats.

Some of the good choices of protein are eggs, peas, tofu and soy foods, beans, lean meats like turkey and chicken, organic dairy products, legumes, and fish as well as seafood. You should pay attention to balancing the macronutrients – protein, carbohydrates, and fats, in your diabetic meal plan to support you with stable blood sugar levels. Fiber, fat, and protein are all slowing down carbohydrate absorption and hence, they enable time for a lower and slower insulin release, along with a steady glucose transport out of the blood and into the targeted tissues.

What Types of Meal Plans or Diet are Recommended for People with Type II Diabetes?

Many dietary patterns are shown to have beneficial effects on insulin resistance. Because multiple models work, people may select the eating patterns that will best work for their condition and overall health. But you will find some commonalities among all the healthy diets or meal plans for diabetic people. All healthy meal plans for people with type II diabetes include limiting red meat and processed sugars, and lots of vegetables. Diabetic people need to have been extra aware of the carb content of their diets, so their blood sugar levels are not increased, or if they are using injectable insulin, they may accurately dose insulin.

Vegetarian or Vegan Diets

A vegan or vegetarian diet may become an excellent choice for diabetic people. Vegan and vegetarian diets are high-carb diets, with around 13% higher carbs as compared to meal plans that include both animal and plant products (which is terrible for diabetes). However, this diet has lower saturated fat and calories commonly, and high fiber, so the associated inflammatory risks of high consumption of meat will be avoided.

A proper vegetarian diet is high in fruits and vegetables, including quality proteins like seeds, beans, and nuts, and plant-based fats like avocado and olive oil. This diet also prioritizes whole grains like quinoa and brown rice instead of refined carbs like processed foods and sweets.

American Diabetes Association (ADA) Diabetes Diet

The ADA diet for diabetic people advocates for a healthy diet, emphasizing balanced energy with exercise IQ. They historically have advocated for most calories that come from complex carbs, which you can get from whole grains like the whole grain cereal and whole grain bread, along with a decreased intake of total fat with majority of them coming from unsaturated fat.

There is no ideal macronutrient ratio and that a dietary plan needs to be individualized. ADA guidelines are advocating for low glycemic index, and avoid beverages IQ that is sweetened with sugar like soda. Fat quality and quantity are important here. Nevertheless, many find these guidelines hard to implement in real life, with the described dietary patterns being more practical and more straightforward for people to manage their meal plan for type II diabetes.

Paleo Diet

The Paleo diet includes eating a moderate amount of protein and has gained so much attention recently. The theory in this dietary pattern is that your genetic background did not evolved in order to meet our modern lifestyle so as to dense limited activity and convenience foods calorically. It also brings us to a hunter-gatherer way of eating, which work better with our physiology. This meal plan is based on fish, eggs, lean meat, nuts, cruciferous and leafy vegetables, fruit, and root vegetables. On the other hand, excluded in this diet are candy, beer, dairy products, soft drinks, refined fats, all kinds of grains, sugar, beans, and any extra salt.

Also, this diet is not specified on caloric intake goals or macronutrient balance. The Paleo diet is lower in total energy, dietary glycemic load, calcium, energy density, carbs, fiber, and saturated fatty acids. But it is higher in dietary cholesterol, unsaturated fatty acids, and some minerals and vitamins. Diabetic people have more stable blood sugar, are less hungry, and they feel better with meal plans that have lower carbs.

Mediterranean Diet

This meal plan for diabetic people is high in vegetables. This is referred to as the true Mediterranean pattern that is traditionally followed in Southern Greece and Italy, and not the Americanized Italian type – those that are heavy in bread and pasta. The Mediterranean diet includes some wine, nuts, some fruits, avocados, lots of fresh vegetables, occasional dairy and meat, fish like sardines, and plant fats like olive oil.

The pattern of eating in this diet is very nutrient-dense, which means that you will be able to get lots of minerals, vitamins, and other healthy nutrients for each consumed calorie. There are 2 versions of Mediterranean diet that are demonstrated to improve diabetes control, including more weight loss and better blood sugar. The 2 versions of this meal plan for diabetic people emphasize either more olive oil or more nuts. Because both versions are beneficial, some Mediterranean meal plans include both of these, such as drizzle zucchini with hemp seeds, oregano, and olive oil or sprinkle chopped almonds on green beans.

5 Diabetes Superfoods to Eat

These are foods that will be beneficial for your health beyond providing fats or calories, carbohydrates, or proteins. Superfoods could be exceptionally rich in kinds of vitamins, or other nutrients that are hugely beneficial for those with type II diabetes.

1. *White balsamic vinegar:* The superfoods vinegar is consumed best as a vinaigrette dressing to your salad, but is beneficial regardless of how you enjoy it. Vinegar is slowing your gastric emptying,

which is helpful for diabetic people. This helps in slowing down your body's glucose release into the bloodstream, enabling for a steady and small insulin response rather than a big insulin surge. This is also increasing satiety. So, if you are enjoying your salad with vinaigrette as your first course, you will be less likely to overeat during your primary course.

2. *Chia seeds:* Chia seed provides protein, omega-3 fatty acids, and fiber. It is a diabetic superfood because it is increasing satiety, bringing down the glycemic load of any meal, and stabilizing the blood sugar. You may add chia seed to your breakfast to keep you full longer. The primary fiber kind in this seed is soluble fiber, turning into a gel when you mix it with water. Chia is fantastic to use in cooking and baking when you need a thickener. When combined with cocoa, low-glycemic index of stevia or agave, and almond milk, chia is a great healthy pudding.

3. *Lentils:* Lentils have great protein, contain essential vitamins, and they have many fibers. This superfood is rich iron and other minerals, and high in B vitamins like the folate. It also has a great balance of complex carbs and protein and is very versatile to partner in your cooking. The brown and green lentils remain firm when they are cooked and they are delicious in salad. On the other hand, the orange lentils get soft when you cook them, which make them suited well in curries, dal, and Indian soups.

4. *Wild salmon:* This superfood is an excellent source of anti-inflammatory omega-3 fatty acids. There are differences in fatty acids between the farmed and wild salmon, due to what the fish eats. The wild salmon is eating smaller fish and they are living in colder waters, causing them to develop higher ratio of anti-inflammatory omega 3s to saturated fats in their meat. Fishes that are farmed are 10x higher in antibiotics, organic pollutants, and other contaminants. These

harmful chemicals are pro-inflammatory and they are associated with increased risk of heart disease and cancer.

5. *Cinnamon:* This is another superfood for people with diabetes, as it lowers their serum glucose, and they are significantly beneficial at doses of 1 tsp per day. Cinnamon is lowering both the postprandial and fasting blood sugar levels. You can sprinkle it on oatmeal, and it is easy to add to any diabetic meal plans. They are also great for coffee. Aside from that, it has high polyphenol content that has added benefit in preventing any health complications.

Foods to be Avoided in Type II Diabetes Meal Plan

Type II diabetic people need to avoid many of the same unhealthy foods that everyone should limit. Included in the dietary restrictions are: refined sugars like cakes, sweets, scones, donuts, candy, cookies, and pastries; sodas, both the diet soda and sugar-sweetened regular soda can increase blood sugar; high-fat animal products like fatty cuts of pork, sausage, red meat, and bacon. Processed carbs like pasta, saltines, and white bread; artificial sweeteners in processed foods with diet label; high-fat dairy products like cream, ice cream, cheese, and whole milk; and trans fats like some salad dressings, bakery products, butter spreads, packaged sauces, and mayonnaise spreads.

Also included are highly processed foods like candies, cookies, chips, and kettle corn; and high fructose corn syrup that can be found in packaged convenience food, soda, and candy. The best way of avoiding these foods is to shop around the edges of your grocery store and take the number of packaged and processed foods minimized in moderation. On the other hand, the best way to eat well for diabetes is to stick with real food in its minimally and whole form. Diabetic people who are eating a healthy meal plan like the ones discussed here can help in reducing the risk of complications of high blood sugar, such as obesity and cardiovascular disease.

Alcohol and Type II Diabetes

For most people who have insulin resistance, the general guideline for moderate consumption of alcohol applies. One glass each day for women and two glasses for men can reduce the risk of cardiovascular disease and it does not have negative impact on diabetes. Nevertheless, alcohol can decrease your blood sugar, and those who have type II diabetes, who are prone to hypoglycemia, especially those who are using insulin, need to be wary of delayed hypoglycemia.

Some of the effective ways to prevent hypoglycemia are alcohol in moderation. Consider eating foods with alcohol drinks to help in minimizing the risk. You may also wear a diabetic alert bracelet so that people would know to offer food when there are hypoglycemic symptoms in you. On the other hand, cocktails and mixed drinks are commonly made with juices or sweeteners and they contain lots of carbs so these drinks can raise your blood sugar levels.

Healthier Choices When Eating Out

Eating out is quite challenging both for the reason that you do not know what exactly a meal would contain when it comes to calories and carbs, and for the reason that eating out with family or friends most commonly result to unintentional pressure of eating the foods that you would be better off without like dessert.

When you eat out, do not hesitate to ask questions about what that particular dish contains or how it has been prepared. You may also look at the menus on the web before going. Furthermore, talk to your family and friends beforehand regarding your reasons to eat healthily. Be open and tell them that these things are essential to your long-term health to stay on your diabetic meal plan and ask them not to encourage to eat things that are not great for you.

Family and friends are usually just trying to show their love by wanting you to enjoy a dessert. They will understand you, and they will eventually support you in your efforts to take care of yourself. Also, when eating out, limit yourself to 2 bites of desserts.

Complications of Type II Diabetes

Insulin resistance may result in several complications like nerve, eye, and kidney damage, and cardiovascular disease. This also means that the cells will not receive the glucose they need for healthy functioning. Good glycemic control will be helpful in preventing long-term complications of insulin resistance. A proper diet to reverse diabetes is also referred to as a medical nutrition therapy for diabetic people.

Conclusion

Reversing diabetes naturally has not been only possible but it is also a preferable solution for modern-day treatment, treating just the signs and symptoms of diabetes without addressing the cause. Reversing diabetes naturally is not about a natural cure or particular home remedy, but solution that involves discussing diet and nutrition. The critical factors on diet and nutrition should be adequately understood, and when adjusted and balanced, may serve to reverse diabetes naturally and successfully and increase the production of your body's insulin. The diet plans and information here will help you understand, prevent, and reverse type II diabetes naturally and successfully.

Final Words

Thank you again for purchasing this book!

I really hope this book is able to help you.

The next step is for you to **join our email newsletter** to receive updates on any upcoming new book releases or promotions. You can sign-up for free and as a bonus, you will also receive our "*7 Fitness Mistakes You Don't Know You're Making*" book! This bonus book breaks down many of the most common fitness mistakes and will demystify many of the complexities and science of getting into shape. Having all this fitness knowledge and science organized into an actionable step-by-step book will help you get started in the right direction in your fitness journey! To join our free email newsletter and grab your free book, please visit the link and signup: **www.hmwpublishing.com/gift**

Finally, if you enjoyed this book, then I would like to ask you for a favor, would you be kind enough to leave a review for this book? It would be greatly appreciated!

Thank you and good luck in your journey!

About the Co-Author

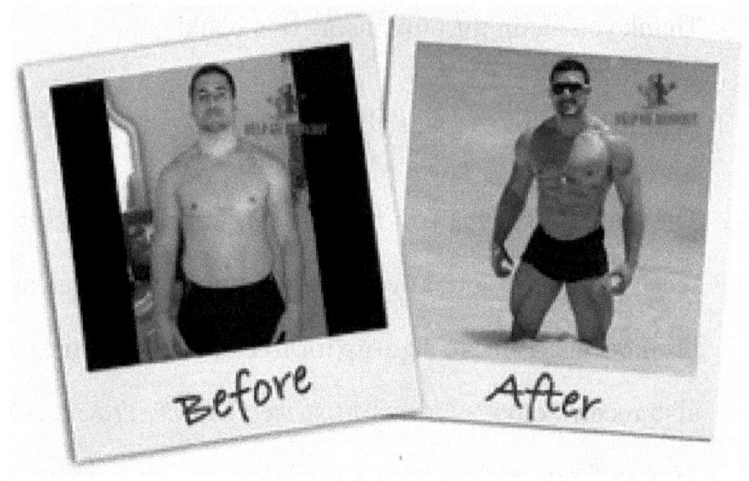

My name is George Kaplo; I'm a certified personal trainer from Montreal, Canada. I'll start off by saying I'm not the biggest guy you will ever meet and this has never really been my goal. In fact, I started working out to overcome my biggest insecurity when I was younger, which was my self-confidence. This was due to my height measuring only 5 foot 5 inches (168cm), it pushed me down to attempt anything I ever wanted to achieve in life. You may be going through some challenges right now, or you may simply want to get fit, and I can certainly relate.

For me personally, I was always kind of interested in the

health & fitness world and wanted to gain some muscle due to the numerous bullying in my teenage years about my height and my overweight body. I figured I couldn't do anything about my height, but I sure can do something about how my body looked like. This was the beginning of my transformation journey. I had no idea where to start, but I just got started. I felt worried and afraid at times that other people would make fun of me for doing the exercises the wrong way. I always wished I had a friend that was next to me who was knowledgeable enough to help me get started and "show me the ropes."

After a lot of work, studying and countless trial and errors. Some people began to notice how I was getting more fit and how I was starting to form a keen interest in the topic. This led many friends and new faces to come to me and ask me for fitness advice. At first, it seemed odd when people asked me to help them get in shape. But what kept me going is when they started to see changes in their own body and told me it's the first time that they saw real results! From there, more people kept coming to me, and it made me realize after so much reading and studying in this field that it did help me but it also allowed me to help others. I'm now a fully certified personal trainer and have trained numerous clients to date who have achieved amazing results.

Today, my brother Alex Kaplo (also a Certified Personal Trainer) and I own & operate this publishing venture, where we bring passionate and expert authors to write about health and fitness topics. We also run an online fitness website "HelpMeWorkout.com" and I would love to connect with by inviting you to visit the website on the following page and signing up to our e-mail newsletter (you will even get a free book). Last but not least, if you are in the position I was once in and you want some guidance, don't hesitate and ask... I'll be there to help you out!

Your friend and coach,

George Kaplo
Certified Personal Trainer

Get another book for Free

I want to thank you for purchasing this book and offer you another book (just as long and valuable as this book), "Health & Fitness Mistakes You Don't Know You're Making", completely free.

Visit the link below to signup and receive it:

www.hmwpublishing.com/gift

In this book, I will break down the most common health & fitness mistakes, you are probably committing right now, and I will reveal how you can easily get in the best shape of your life!

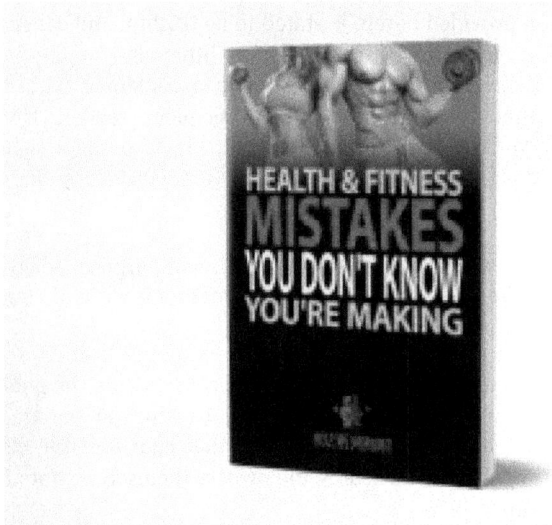

In addition to this valuable gift, you will also have an opportunity to get our new books for free, enter giveaways, and receive other valuable emails from me. Again, visit the link to sign up:

www.hmwpublishing.com/gift

Copyright 2017 by HMW Publishing - All Rights Reserved.

This document by HMW Publishing owned by the A&G Direct Inc company, is geared towards providing exact and reliable information in regards to the topic and issue covered. The publication is sold with the idea that the publisher is not required to render accounting, officially permitted, or otherwise, qualified services. If advice is necessary, legal or professional, a practiced individual in the profession should be ordered.

From a Declaration of Principles which was accepted and approved equally by a Committee of the American Bar Association and a Committee of Publishers and Associations.

In no way is it legal to reproduce, duplicate, or transmit any part of this document in either electronic means or in printed format. Recording of this publication is strictly prohibited, and any storage of this document is not allowed unless with written permission from the publisher. All rights reserved.

The information provided herein is stated to be truthful and consistent, in that any liability, in terms of inattention or otherwise, by any usage or abuse of any policies, processes, or directions contained within is the solitary and utter responsibility of the recipient reader. Under no circumstances will any legal responsibility or blame be held against the publisher for any reparation, damages, or monetary loss due to the information herein, either directly or indirectly.

The information herein is offered for informational purposes solely, and is universal as so. The presentation of the information is without contract or any type of guarantee assurance.

The trademarks that are used are without any consent, and the publication of the trademark is without permission or backing by the trademark owner. All trademarks and brands within this book are for clarifying purposes only and are the owned by the owners themselves, not affiliated with this document.

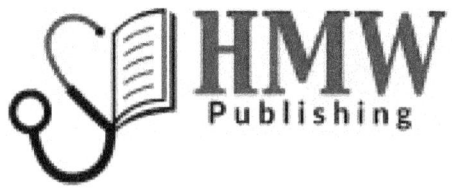

For more great books visit:

HMWPublishing.com

www.ingramcontent.com/pod-product-compliance
Lightning Source LLC
Chambersburg PA
CBHW070033040426
42333CB00040B/1668